Managing Chronic Pain with Opioids in Primary Care

SECOND EDITION

Kevin L. Zacharoff, MD
Director of Medical Affairs
Inflexxion, Inc.
Newton, Massachusetts

Bill H. McCarberg, MD
Assistant Clinical Professor of Medicine
University of California, San Diego, School of Medicine
San Diego, California
Founder, Chronic Pain Management Program
Kaiser Permanente
San Diego, California

Lori Reisner, PharmD, FCSHP
Associate Clinical Professor of Pharmacy
University of California, San Francisco, School of Pharmacy
UCSF Medical Center
San Francisco, California

Synne Wing Venuti, MSW
Product Manager
Inflexxion, Inc.
Newton, Massachusetts

Inflexxion®, Inc.
320 Needham Street, Suite 100
Newton, MA 02464

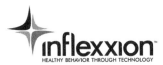

Inflexxion®, Inc.
320 Needham Street, Suite 100
Newton, MA 02464
www.inflexxion.com

Disclaimer

The information provided is not medical advice provided by a physician and is not a substitute for such advice. This guide contains recommendations compiled by clinicians in the field to assist others caring for chronic pain patients. We define chronic pain as persistent pain that has lasted for more than 3 months. Clinicians should use their best judgment on how to incorporate information from this guide into their daily practice. If users of the guide have any questions or concerns regarding usage, they should seek the advice of a licensed physician.

Acknowledgments

Supported by an educational grant from Endo Pharmaceuticals, Inc, Chadds Ford, PA.

First Edition funded in part by the Massachusetts Department of Public Health under a grant from the Bureau of Justice Assistance.

We would like to thank Steven Passik, PhD, for permission to reproduce part of the PADT tool and Howard A. Heit, MD, FACP, FASAM for permission to include his Medication Safety Agreement.

Produced by Silverchair Science + Communications, Inc., 316 East Main Street, Charlottesville, Virginia 22902
Printed in the United States of America

ISBN- 0-9825298-0-5

Contents

Preface

The purpose of this pocket guide is to provide primary care clinicians with a user-friendly, logically organized, and comprehensive manual for the evaluation and treatment of patients who might benefit from opioid analgesia. It addresses clinicians' concerns about prescribing opioids, while providing for the safe and effective treatment of patients who have moderate to severe chronic pain.

This pocket guide includes the following material:

- Evidence-based information about assessing the risk of opioid abuse
- How to prevent or manage opioid-related adverse effects
- When and how to discontinue opioid treatment
- Practical tips on how to organize a practice to support the safe prescribing of opioids
- How to limit the likelihood of aberrant drug-related behavior

The first part of the guide provides general information about the assessment and long-term management of chronic pain patients with opioids. This section is followed by a series of appendices. The appendices contain detailed how-to information, along with examples of some commonly used tools that can help to determine a particular patient's risk for misusing or abusing his/her opioid prescription.

This guide is small enough to carry with you when seeing patients in the clinical setting, and it provides easy access to information regarding specific opioid-related questions. We hope that you will find this reference useful.

Kevin L. Zacharoff, MD
Bill H. McCarberg, MD
Lori Reisner, PharmD, FCSHP
Synne Wing Venuti, MSW

Safely Managing Chronic Pain with Opioids

Optimal treatment of patients with moderate to severe chronic pain presents a number of challenges for physicians and other health care providers in primary care:

- It may not always be clear when an opioid analgesic is an appropriate component of the pain treatment plan.
- If opioids are indicated, important issues to address include:
  - Which medications are optimal for a specific pain problem?
  - What should be done if the medication is not well tolerated?
  - How should the patient be monitored?
  - How long should the patient be treated?

The basis for the long-term use of opioids in the treatment of cancer pain has been fairly well established. Alternatively, a variety of controversies and differences of opinion have surrounded the use of opioid therapy when treating chronic *noncancer* pain. Issues range from the scientific basis for efficacy (safe and appropriate use), to health care providers' fears of legislative reprimand for indiscriminate prescribing. Among the most significant of the controversies is the abuse and misuse of opioids: Their use has increased substantially since 1990, along with a rising mortality rate from these aberrant behaviors.

Primary care clinicians and specialists alike require evidence-based recommendations for the safe and appropriate use of opioids in treating this significant patient population. As a result, they have looked to respected pain management experts and societies for guidance.

In response to this need, the American Pain Society (APS), in partnership with the American Academy of Pain Medicine (AAPM), commissioned a yearlong, multidisciplinary panel to develop evidence-based guidelines on chronic opioid therapy in adults with noncancer pain, released in 2009.[1] These guidelines are based on a comprehensive and systematic review of published evidence on the subject. Most important, these guidelines are targeted toward both primary care and specialty settings. The panel hopes to reach "all clinicians who provide care for adults with chronic noncancer pain, including cancer survivors with chronic pain due to their cancer or its treatment."

Summary of Topics and Recommendations Adapted from American Pain Society and American Academy of Pain Medicine Joint Guidelines

1. **Patient Selection and Risk Stratification**
   a. A detailed history and physical examination
   b. Assessment of the risk of likelihood of abuse, misuse, or addiction (*Proper patient selection is critical. It requires a comprehensive benefit-to-harm evaluation that weighs the potential positive effects of opioids on pain and function against potential risks.* **Thorough risk assessment and stratification is appropriate in every case.**)

2. **Informed Consent and Opioid Management Plans**
   a. Informed consent for opioid therapy should include items that any informed consent would normally contain:
      i. Goals of treatment
      ii. Expectations
      iii. Risks and alternatives
   b. A written opioid management plan should be considered. (For more information about opioid agreements and a sample agreement, please visit *http://www.PainEDU.org.*)

3. Initiation and Titration of Chronic Opioid Therapy
Initial treatment should *always* be individually determined, and used as a trial of therapy—not a definitive course of treatment.

4. Use of Methadone
It is recommended that methadone be used *only* by clinicians familiar with its use and risks.

5. Monitoring Patients
Periodic reassessment is paramount and includes documentation of:
a. Level of function
b. Progress toward predetermined goals
c. Presence of adverse events
d. Compliance (or lack of)

6. High-Risk Patients
High-risk patients should only be treated by clinicians (such as mental health or addiction specialists) who are able to implement more frequent and stringent monitoring approaches.

7. Dose Escalations, High-Dose Opioid Therapy, Opioid Rotation, and Indications for Discontinuation of Therapy
a. When repeated escalations are necessary, consider the potential causes for this increased need as well as the risks and benefits.
b. Increased vigilance (such as more frequent follow-up visits) should be considered in patients on high-dose opioid therapy.
c. Opioid rotation should be considered for issues such as tolerance of adverse effects or unsatisfactory efficacy.
d. Discontinuation (tapering or weaning) of opioid therapy is recommended for patients who repeatedly engage in aberrant drug-related behaviors.

8. Opioid-Related Adverse Effects
Common adverse effects need to be anticipated and appropriately addressed.

9. **Use of Psychotherapeutic Co-Interventions**

   Interventions such as cognitive-behavioral therapy (along with other interdisciplinary therapies and other adjunctive nonopioid therapies) should be routinely integrated into long-term opioid treatment.

10. **Driving and Work Safety**

    Counsel patients about transient or lasting cognitive impairment.

11. **Identifying a Medical Home and When to Obtain Consultation**

    a. A clinician needs to be identified as the person with primary responsibility for the patient's overall medical care. This clinician may or may not be the one prescribing the patient's chronic opioid therapy, but should coordinate consultation (and all communication) between all disciplines involved in the patient's care.

    b. Consultation should be considered as in any other situation: when the clinician feels that the patient may benefit from other resources beyond his or her capability.

12. **Breakthrough Pain**

    Patients on around-the-clock therapy may need prn opioids, and their use should always be based on a risk-benefit analysis.

13. **Opioids in Pregnancy**

    a. As in other situations, clinicians should counsel women of childbearing capacity about the risks and benefits of chronic opioid therapy during and after pregnancy. In most situations, opioid use during pregnancy should be discouraged or minimized, unless benefits are determined to outweigh the risks.

    b. In the event that chronic opioid therapy is used during pregnancy, the needs of the mother and the baby must be appropriately anticipated.

14. Opioid Policies

Clinicians *must* be aware of policies about the medical use of chronic opioids for the treatment of patients' noncancer pain. These policies include:

a. Federal laws

b. State laws

c. Regulatory guidelines

d. Policy statements

These guidelines may seem quite simplistic if taken individually. Their true significance, however, is their purpose as part of a formulated plan for safe and appropriate use of opioids in this important population of patients. Very often, patients with noncancer pain are denied the appropriate course of treatment or quantity of therapeutic agent; this is the result of a strategic plan deficit in approaching the long-term treatment of chronic pain with opioids. If used in their complete form, federal and state laws, guidelines, and policies can do much to improve the quality of care of these patients and to increase the comfort level of clinicians. Coupled with good clinical judgment, these recommendations can provide clinicians with the framework for safer use of opioids and more efficacious care of patients with chronic noncancer pain; the guidelines can also minimize the risk associated with opioid use.

Clinicians may be reluctant to prescribe opioids because they are increasingly concerned about the possibility of causing opioid addiction in some individuals; they are also apprehensive that regulatory agencies may accuse them of inappropriate prescribing.

The federal government attempts to ensure the availability of opioid analgesics for legitimate medical and scientific purposes, while controlling the abuse and illegal diversion of such substances. The U.S. Food and Drug Administration (FDA) is charged with the task of approving medications that are deemed as safe and effective for medical use. Once approved by the FDA, a drug may be prescribed as labeled, or in an "off-label" manner, at the prescribing clinician's discretion; such use is based on a therapeutic risk-benefit evaluation and conformity to community standards of good medical practice.

In 2002, Congress reauthorized the *Prescription Drug User Fee Act* (PDUFA III). One of the goals of the PDUFA was to produce guidance for the pharmaceutical industry on risk management activities for drug and biological products. The intent of the FDA was to create a plan that would encompass the idea of ***medication risk management.***

Specifically, the FDA describes medication risk management as an iterative four-part process that should be continuous throughout a medication's lifecycle; the results of risk assessment should inform the manufacturer's further decisions regarding risk minimization:

1. Assessing a medication's benefit-risk balance
2. Developing and implementing tools to minimize risks while preserving benefits
3. Evaluating tool effectiveness and reassessing the benefit-risk balance
4. Making adjustments, as appropriate, to the risk minimization tools to further improve the benefit-risk balance

Within the context of medication risk management, the FDA may require the manufacturer to submit a *Risk Minimization Action Plan* (RiskMAP) as part of the FDA's application for approval.

Risk Minimization Action Plans (RiskMAPs)

The FDA defines a RiskMAP as the *"strategic safety program designed to meet specific goals and objectives in minimizing known risks of a medication while preserving its benefits."* For the majority of FDA-approved products, the labeling and routine reporting requirements of adverse events are sufficient to mitigate risks and preserve benefits. A RiskMAP is required in a relatively small number of cases when additional measures are deemed necessary to ensure that the benefits of a drug outweigh the risks. The intent of a submitted RiskMAP is to lay out a plan (processes or systems) to minimize known safety risks, including risks of adverse effects, aberrant drug-related behaviors, and negative outcomes relative to the risk. The submitted plan is to include such processes as:

1. Targeted education and outreach to health care practitioners or patients, to communicate risks and appropriate safety behaviors
2. Reminder systems, processes, or forms to foster reduced-risk prescribing and use
3. Performance-linked access systems that guide the prescribing, dispensing, and use of the product; these systems target the population and conditions of use most likely to confer benefits and to minimize particular risks

Decisions by the FDA to require a RiskMAP continue today on a case-by-case basis; these decisions are based on the agency's own interpretation of risk information.

In September 2007, the President signed the *Food and Drug Administration Amendments Act of 2007* (FDAAA) into law. This new law (H.R. 3580) represents a **significant addition to FDA authority.** Among the many components of the FDAAA law, the PDUFA (which was expiring) was reauthorized and expanded. The resulting law contained numerous provisions designed to:

- Better inform the public about drug safety.
- Provide new tools for the FDA to reduce risks and unsafe drug use.

Risk Evaluation and Mitigation Strategies (REMS)

The passage of the FDAAA:

- Enhanced the FDA's authority to require drug labeling changes and additional post-market studies.
- Gave the FDA the authority to require *Risk Evaluation and Mitigation Strategies* (REMS) for new products *and* already-approved products; REMS may be required if the FDA becomes aware of new safety information and determines that

a REMS is necessary to "ensure the benefits of the drug outweigh the risks of the drug."

- REMS expand on the assessment of medication risk management (previously built into RiskMAPs) to include periodic reassessment and modification as necessary.
- Contents of REMS include:
  - A medication guide
  - A patient package insert, if such an insert may help to mitigate a serious risk of the drug
  - Elements to assure safe use of the medication
  - A communication plan to convey information to health care providers that supports the mitigation strategy
- Grants the FDA the authority to require additional post-approval studies. If marketed medications are found to be associated with new potential risks, the FDA can require labeling changes or additional research to address these risks.
- Stopped short of requiring REMS for all new drugs, as was originally proposed. The FDA will therefore decide on a case-by-case basis whether a drug that is pending approval warrants a REMS.

Manufacturers that fail to make FDA-requested labeling changes, or to conduct timely post-market studies, would be found in violation of the FDAAA and subject to fines. Pharmaceutical companies could also be penalized for failing to implement a requested, submitted, and approved REMS.

The FDAAA, REMS, and the use of chronic opioid therapy pain management crossed paths in early 2009: At that time, the FDA sent letters to manufacturers of all extended-release opioid drugs, indicating that these drugs will be required to have a REMS in addition to their RiskMAPs. This measure would be taken to ensure that the benefits of the drugs continue to outweigh the risks of:

1. Use of certain opioid products in non–opioid-tolerant individuals
2. Abuse
3. Overdose, both *accidental and intentional*

The FDA stated in this letter that:

- "The agency has long been concerned about adverse events associated with this class of drug and has taken steps in cooperation with drug manufacturers to address these risks. We intend to use the agency's REMS authority under the Food and Drug Administration Amendments Act of 2007 (FDAAA) to mitigate the risks of these drugs."
- "Opioid drugs have benefit when used properly and are a necessary component of pain management for certain patients."
- "Opioid drugs have serious risks when used improperly."
- "The FDA, drug manufacturers, and others have taken a number of steps in the past to prevent misuse, abuse, and accidental overdose of these drugs, including providing additional warnings in product labeling, implementing a risk management plan (RiskMAP), conducting inter-agency collaborations, and issuing direct communications to both prescribers and patients."
- "Despite these efforts, the rates of misuse and abuse, and of accidental overdose of opioids, have risen over the past decade."
- "The FDA believes that establishing a REMS for opioids will reduce these risks, while still ensuring that patients with legitimate need for these drugs will continue to have appropriate access."
- "The REMS would be intended to ensure that the benefits of these drugs continue to outweigh certain risks."

All companies that make extended-release opioids have been asked by the FDA to work together, as opposed to separately, to create a single, broad-application REMS program that will encompass all extended-release medications in this class. Although individual medications have been required to submit a REMS as part of their application, or to implement one post–FDA approval, this is the first time that the FDA has indicated that a REMS will be needed on a class-wide basis. The likely impetus is the number of drug-related deaths associated with extended-release opioids.

Once a clear direction exists, the FDA will likely consult with the Drug Enforcement Administration (DEA) on the class-wide REMS. The Controlled Substances Act, and DEA regulations that require manufacturers and registrants of controlled substances to maintain effective controls against diversion and compliance with REMS, could arguably be viewed as a part of this duty. Drug manufacturers will need to consider that the DEA will evaluate compliance with REMS as a factor in determining ongoing compliance with DEA requirements.

Clinical Implications

If REMS are required for extended-release opioids, there will be a need to provide mechanisms to ensure safe use of these medications. These mechanisms should ensure that *prescribers, dispensers*, and *patients* are all aware of and understand the risks and appropriate use of these products.

There is little doubt that the finalized program will have requirements with some degree of clinical impact at all stakeholder levels:

- Ongoing, opioid-specific training (and possibly certification) for clinicians and pharmacists
- A higher level of clinician vigilance than previously required
- Expanded use of doctor-patient opioid agreements:
  - Detailing the responsibilities of both clinician and patient
  - Including review and confirmation of patient comprehension of the medication guide for the specific medication
  - Providing information about the safe and appropriate use of opioid medications, and the dangers of sharing medications
- A plan that outlines continued monitoring of these initiatives to ensure that the goals are being met

The challenge will be to provide access to extended-release opioids for appropriate patients in need, while achieving the desired goals.

Useful Tips for Safe and Appropriate Use of Chronic Opioid Therapy

- Select patients carefully and assess opioid risk.
- Obtain informed consent and use an opioid agreement.
- Consider initial treatment only as a *trial* of therapy.
- Only use methadone if you are familiar with its use and associated risks.
- Monitor patients periodically and as warranted by your opioid risk assessment.
- Consider consultation with a specialist in high-risk patients.
- Carefully titrate opioid dose to effect and consider opioid rotation when appropriate.
- Monitor the patient closely for adverse effects.
- Consider an integrated approach to pain management with other disciplines (e.g., cognitive-behavioral therapy).
- Include a methodology that allows for the treatment of breakthrough pain.
- Have an exit strategy.

Suggested Readings

Chou R, Fanciullo GJ, Fine PG, et al. Clinical guidelines for the use of chronic opioid therapy in chronic noncancer pain. *J Pain* 2009; 10(2):113–130.

Model Policy for the Use of Controlled Substances for the Treatment of Pain. Federation of State Medical Boards of the United States, Inc. Adopted as policy by the House of Delegates of the Federation of State Medical Boards of the United States, Inc., May 2004.

The Comprehensive Drug Abuse Prevention and Control Act of 1970, Pub. L. No. 91-513, 84 Stat. 1236 (Oct. 27, 1970).

Federal Register / Vol. 74, No. 74 / Monday, April 20, 2009 / Notices Department of Health and Human Services Food and Drug Administration [Docket No. FDA–2009–N–0143] *Risk Evaluation and Mitigation Strategies for Certain Opioid Drugs*; Notice of Public Meeting.

Gourlay DL, Heit HA, Almahrez A. Universal precautions in pain medicine: a rational approach to the treatment of chronic pain. *Pain Medicine* 2205;6(2):107–112.

Preparing Your Practice

There are many steps to consider when preparing your practice for the multiple regulatory issues and responsibilities of prescribing an opioid for pain treatment.

- Go to your state medical board's Web site, and review state laws regarding opioid treatment.
  - A summary of state regulations is available at *http://www.painpolicy.wisc.edu/domestic/state_profiles/index.html*.
- Know the status of your state's prescription monitoring program.
- *Achieving Balance in Federal and State Pain Policy: A Guide to Evaluation,* 5th ed., provides a state-by-state listing of classification schedules, drugs covered, and type of program (electronic, triplicate, etc). See *http://www.painpolicy.wisc.edu/Achieving_Balance/EG2008.pdf*
- Understand your legal responsibility:
  - Review the U.S. Department of Justice Drug Enforcement Administration's overview of the Controlled Substances Act at *http://www.deadiversion.usdoj.gov/schedules/*.
  - Familiarize yourself with legal/regulatory compliance issues.
  - For more information, go to *http://www.legalsideofpain.com* and *http://www.painpolicy.wisc.edu*.
- Familiarize yourself with common characteristics of patients at risk for opioid abuse (see Appendix 5).
- Educate your office staff (see Appendix 1).
- Develop and implement compliance programs for:
  - Pain management billing and coding
  - The use of controlled substances to treat pain
  - The office-based treatment of opioid addiction

Initial Patient Assessment for Opioid Therapy

The guidelines below focus on elements of the patient assessment that are specifically relevant to long-term opioid therapy. The main goals of patient assessment for opioid therapy are as follows:

- To determine whether opioids are the most appropriate treatment for the patient, or whether treatments with different risk-benefit ratios should be considered
- To triage the patient into levels of risk for substance abuse
- To inform an assessment of the risk-benefit ratio of long-term opioid therapy

Essential features of the patient assessment for opioid therapy that are identical to features in all other patient assessments in medicine (see Appendix 6 for details):

- Chief complaint
- History of present illness
  - Pain history
  - Pain medication history
- Past history, including psychiatric and substance abuse histories of both the patient *and* his or her family
- Social history
- Family history
- Physical examination
  - Features relevant to pain and to substance abuse
- Additional information
  - Urine medication monitoring
  - Blood tests

- Screening for risk of substance abuse
- Prescription monitoring report
- Outside medical records

Note: It is assumed that an appropriate evaluation for the underlying pain complaint is conducted with attention to the underlying diagnosis and any primary treatment (e.g., cancer or infection).

Assessing Risk

The clinician can assess risk of abuse and addiction by observing the patient's behavior and eliciting information during the initial evaluation and subsequent visits.

- Appendix 5 lists some behaviors that have been associated with addiction.
- Assessing risk is not an exact science:
  - When in doubt, get a consultation from a pain or addiction specialist or refer the patient.

Screener and Opioid Assessment for Patients with Pain

The Screener and Opioid Assessment for Patients with Pain (SOAPP®) is a simple, validated, paper-and-pencil self-report tool that provides a score for clinicians to assess risk *before* prescribing an opioid (see Appendix 7). The SOAPP is **not intended** to rule out opioid therapy as a possible option for treating chronic pain. Rather, the SOAPP score, along with other clinical findings, can help the provider make a risk-benefit assessment regarding the use of opioid therapy. If opioid therapy is determined to be an appropriate treatment option, the SOAPP can help the provider determine the necessary level of monitoring to safely prescribe long-term opioid therapy for a given patient (see Appendix 7).

- Available versions of the SOAPP:
  - SOAPP (Version 1.0, 24-item)
  - 14-item SOAPP
  - 5-item SOAPP (SOAPP-SF)
  - 24-item SOAPP-R (Revised Version)
- In summary, the SOAPP:
  - Identifies risk level of patients for both documentation *and* treatment planning

- Is **not** intended to rule out patients for opioid therapy
- Is part of a multifaceted approach to risk assessment
■ Please see *http://www.PainEDU.org* for more information about the SOAPP, including instructions and scoring. You may also view the tutorial at the site or download the tool.

Current Opioid Misuse Measure

The Current Opioid Misuse Measure (COMM)® is a brief, validated, paper-and-pencil patient self-assessment, intended to help clinicians identify whether a patient who is *currently on long-term opioid therapy* may be exhibiting aberrant behaviors associated with opioid medication misuse. The COMM is **not intended** to rule out opioid therapy as a possible treatment option for treating chronic pain. Rather, the COMM score (along with other clinical findings) can help the provider make a risk-benefit assessment regarding the continued use of opioid therapy. If long-term opioid therapy is determined to be an appropriate treatment option, the COMM can help the provider determine the necessary level of monitoring (see Appendix 8).

The COMM:

■ Includes 17 items
■ Is simple to score
■ Is usually completed in less than 10 minutes
■ Was validated with a group of approximately 500 chronic pain patients on opioid therapy
■ In summary, the COMM:
- Identifies the risk level of patients for both documentation *and* treatment planning
- Is **not** intended to rule out patients for opioid therapy
- Is part of a multifaceted approach to risk assessment
■ Please see *http://www.PainEDU.org* for more information about the COMM, including instructions and scoring. You may also view the tutorial at the site or download the tool.

Triage Guide

This table provides criteria for assigning a risk level and determining the next steps for your patient.

Risk Level	Characteristics	Management
Low	No history of substance abuse; minimal if any risk factors*	Can be managed by primary care physician
		If aberrant behaviors are observed, consider increasing risk category
Medium	History of substance abuse (not prescription opioid abuse); significant risk factors*	Primary care physician co-manages with addiction and/or pain specialists
	Patient previously assigned to low-risk category; exhibits aberrant behaviors†	If aberrant behaviors are observed or persist, consider assigning to high-risk category
High	Active substance abuse problem; history of prescription opioid abuse	Opioids may not be appropriate in the primary care setting
	Patient previously assigned to medium-risk category; exhibits aberrant behaviors	Refer patient to specialists in management of patients with comorbid pain and addictive disorders
		Continue to manage patient's medical care and monitor specialized care

*Risk factors for prescription opioid abuse include active substance abuse, past substance abuse, family history of substance abuse, history of prescription drug abuse,

(notes continue on next page)

current or past mental health disorder (personal or family), younger age, and criminal activity. None of these risks is absolute, and opioid addiction may occur in their absence.

†See Appendices 5 and 14 for lists of aberrant behaviors.

Initiate Opioid Trial

Opioid Trial Initiation Checklist

- Physicians:
  - *Always* **consider opioid therapy to be a trial of therapy**
  - Select appropriate opioid (see Appendix 13)
- Office staff:
  - Ensure that patient's chart includes:
    - Completed opioid agreement (see Appendix 17)
    - Medication flow chart (see Appendix 2)

Patient Medication Agreements

- A patient medication agreement (sometimes referred to as an opioid "contract") *along with* informed consent establishes clear expectations between physician and patient. It specifies:
  - Purpose of opioid therapy
  - Side effects
  - Treatment goals
  - Physician's role in responsible opioid prescribing
  - Patient's role in responsible opioid use
- Patient should review and sign the medication agreement after the initial assessment and, if possible, *before* an opioid trial is initiated.
- See Appendix 17 or go to *http://www.PainEDU.org* for sample patient medication agreements.

Key Components of a Patient Medication Agreement

- Opioid prescriptions are provided by only one primary care physician (PCP).
- Patients agree not to ask for opioid medications from any other health care provider without the knowledge and assent of the PCP.

- Patients agree to keep all scheduled medical appointments.
- Patients agree to provide urine samples for drug screens as requested.
- No prescriptions will be refilled early.
- No prescriptions will be refilled if lost, destroyed, or if medication has been stolen.
- Prescription refills will be authorized only during regular office hours.
- Patients agree to comply fully with all aspects of the treatment program, including behavioral medicine (psychology/psychiatry) and physical therapy if recommended.

Patient Education

When initiating opioid therapy, clinicians should always carefully describe the rationale for the use of these medications, including the potential side effects and how to minimize them. Patients frequently have concerns about becoming addicted to the medication or being perceived by friends or family as being an addict. For these and a number of other reasons, compliance with opioid treatment will likely be improved when clinicians spend the time to address patient concerns.

For patient medication safety resources, patients may be referred to *http://www.painaction.com*.

Choosing an Opioid

Depending on their pain profile, past experience, and abuse risk, some patients with chronic pain are best treated with:

- A long-acting opioid on a fixed-dose schedule for background pain, and a short-acting opioid for breakthrough pain
- A long-acting opioid only
- A short-acting opioid only

Long-Acting Opioids

- Slower onset of action (30–90 minutes)
- Relatively long duration (4–72 hours)
- Used on an around-the-clock basis for patients with constant background pain
- Long-acting by virtue of:
  - Intrinsic pharmacokinetic properties such as:
    - Methadone
    - Levorphanol
  - Incorporation into a slow-release delivery system such as:
    - Controlled-release morphine
    - Controlled-release tramadol
    - Controlled-release oxycodone
    - Transdermal fentanyl
    - Controlled-release oxymorphone

Short-Acting Opioids

- Fast onset of action (10–60 minutes)
- Short duration of action (2–4 hours)
- Used for patients with intermittent pain or breakthrough episodes that are superimposed on constant background pain such as:
  - Codeine

- Hydrocodone
- Hydromorphone
- Oxycodone
- Tramadol
- Fentanyl (available for transmucosal use as a "lollipop" or as a rapid-dissolving buccal formulation)

Combination Products

- Combine an opioid with a nonopioid analgesic (acetaminophen or a nonsteroidal anti-inflammatory drug [NSAID]).
- Used for patients who do not require dose escalation beyond the limits of the nonopioid component.
- Combining different products generally gives better results than using either product alone.

Selected Combination Drugs

Opioid	Combined with Acetaminophen	Combined with Ibuprofen
Codeine	✓	
Hydrocodone	✓	✓
Oxycodone	✓	✓

Abuse-Deterrent Formulations of Opioids

Medications with abuse potential, such as prescription opioid medications, should be readily available to people who need them. As concern continues to rise with regard to opioid misuse and abuse, there is renewed interest in the development of abuse-deterrent formulations of opioids. "Abuse-deterrent" generally refers to the ability of the drug formulation to *restrict or reduce the potential for abuse* of the drug through a variety of different approaches, including physical and chemical strategies.

Physical Approaches to Deterrence

This strategy may also be referred to as "tamper-resistant," by preventing the physical manipulation and ultimate extraction of the medication, for nonmedical use, or by reducing ingestion by alternate routes such as:

- Smoking
- Snorting
- Chewing
- Crushing
- Injecting
- Inhaling

This type of formulation may not decrease abuse or misuse of the original formulation by the originally intended route of administration (e.g., oral).

Chemical Approaches to Deterrence

- Agonist-antagonist formulations
  - This refers to opioids that are combined with opioid antagonists for the purpose of deterring abuse. The antagonist is either present in subclinical quantities, and only exerts effects when large enough doses are consumed; or is poorly absorbed by oral routes; or is released as the result of tampering with the formulation.
- Combination formulations with aversive compounds
  - This refers to compounding opioids with agents that have chemically irritating or unpleasant properties. If swallowed, they would normally have no effect (e.g., capsaicin), but upon snorting, injecting, or inhaling, they would promote intense discomfort and burning, or uncomfortable symptoms (e.g., niacin), such as flushing or "hot flashes."
- Other mechanisms
  - Alternative forms of application, such as transdermal preparations

■ Use of "pro-drug" compounds that only exert a therapeutic effect after some degree of metabolism

Abuse-deterrent opioid formulations may play a significant role in curbing prescribed opioid abuse and misuse. They may have the potential to deliver an opioid when appropriate, but limit abuse and misuse. These formulations may help to reduce the public health burden of prescription opioid abuse, and also make it easier for clinicians to prescribe them when they are the appropriate choice to manage chronic pain. After validation of their ability to live up to expectations, they may become the new generation of opioids and make nondeterrent formulations of opioids obsolete.

Recommended Starting Doses of Opioids

■ Caution should be used in initiating opioids in patients who are not currently taking opioids.
■ Respiratory depression can occur.
■ For opioid-naïve patients, start with low doses of opioid and titrate up until pain relief is obtained without unacceptable toxicity.
■ See Appendix 13 for dosing recommendations by medication.

Follow-Up Checklist

- Use the Follow-Up Visit Form to record information (see Appendix 14).
- Review medication flow chart; take pill counts.
  - Medication flow charts can identify early refills.
  - Pill and/or patch counts can help identify whether patients are using their medications inappropriately.
- Perform a physical examination and take a comprehensive history.
  - Evaluate the location and aggravating physical characteristics of the pain; determine if there has been a change since the last visit.
  - Conduct mental health assessment at least annually (see Appendix 9).
- Conduct periodic urine medication monitoring (see Appendix 10) or other toxicology screens and other relevant laboratory tests.
  - Conduct endocrine laboratory tests annually (see Appendix 10).
- Determine if brief intervention is needed for possible substance abuse (see Appendix 11).
- Determine the action plan:*
  - Continue present opioid regimen
  - Adjust regimen as follows:
    - Add/adjust concomitant therapy: _____
    - Add/adjust nonpharmacologic therapy: _____
    - Adjust present opioid: _____
    - Rotate opioid: _____
  - Exit strategy: Taper patient off opioid regimen
  - Other: _____

*Adapted from Pain Assessment and Documentation Tool (PADT), courtesy of Steven Passik, PhD, Associate Attending Psychologist, Memorial Sloan-Kettering Cancer Center, New York, NY.

Preventing and Managing Side Effects

Side Effect	Prevention	Treatment
Confusion	For high-risk (e.g., Alzheimer's) patients maximize nonopioid regimen	Lower dose; rotate to another opioid; low-dose neuroleptics if necessary
Constipation	Stool softeners; bowel stimulants; non-pharmacologic measures	Use common measures to treat constipation or rotate to another opioid
Dizziness	—	Antivertiginous agents (e.g., scopolamine); lower dose (if possible); add co-analgesics
Edema and sweating	—	Rotate to another opioid
Endocrine dysfunction/ reduced libido/hypogonadism	Assess endocrine status at baseline and at least annually thereafter	Consider opioid rotation; consider strategies that allow opioid dose reduction; testosterone supplementation if hypogonadism is diagnosed; consider consultation with an endocrinologist; monitor prostate-specific antigen in males on testosterone supplementation

(continued)

Side Effect	Prevention	Treatment
Hives	If patient has history, use opioid in different chemical group or family	Rotate to another opioid; symptomatic treatment
Myoclonus	—	Rotate to another opioid; to suppress myoclonus, consider low doses of baclofen, clonazepam, or gabapentin
Nausea	Co-prescribe anti-emetic if patient has history of opioid-induced nausea/vomiting	Rotate to another opioid
Pruritus	—	Rotate to another opioid; antihistamines
Rash	If patient has history, use opioid in different chemical group or family	Rotate to another opioid; symptomatic treatment
Respiratory depression	"Start low, go slow." Start with low doses of opioid and titrate to effect; monitor patient closely	Close observation, supportive measures (airway, breathing, and circulation, or "ABC"); naloxone for overdose with respiratory or hemo-dynamic compromise
Sedation	"Start low, go slow." Start with low doses of opioid and titrate to effect; monitor patient closely	Lower dose (if possible); add co-analgesics; add stimulants

(continued)

Side Effect	Prevention	Treatment
Urinary retention	—	Rotate to another opioid; lower dose (if possible)
Vomiting	Co-prescribe anti-emetics with each regimen if patient has history	Rotate to another opioid; antiemetic

Note: These symptoms, even though present in patients on opioid therapy, may be due to other causes; a diagnostic evaluation is *always* recommended.

Data from Zacharoff KZ, Pujol LM, Corsini E. *The PainEDU.org Manual: A Pocket Guide to Pain Management,* 4th ed. Newton, MA: Inflexxion®, Inc. Available at *http://www.painEDU.org.*

Opioid Rotation

Clinical Rationale for Changing an Opioid

Patients have been shown to respond to opioids differently based on a number of different variables, including genetic predisposition. This provides a rationale to rotate (switch) to a different opioid in the event that patient response does not yield successful management of the painful condition. In some cases, rotation may be necessary more than one time or even a number of times to find the right opioid. Below are some reasons to support the strategy of opioid rotation.

Lack of Efficacy

- Development of opioid analgesic tolerance
- Poor response to first-line opioid
- Inability to tolerate effective dose
- Dose required to produce analgesia exceeds maximum daily dose recommendations (*although treatment should always be individualized*)

Development of Intolerable Side Effects

- Gastrointestinal (e.g., constipation, nausea, vomiting)
- Central nervous system (e.g., sedation, somnolence, dysphoria, hallucinations, myoclonus)
- Cardiovascular (e.g., orthostatic hypotension)

Change in Patient Status

- Inability to swallow
- Poor peripheral vascular status/poor absorption of transdermal medications
- Patient is NPO

■ Requirement of high-dose opioids that cannot be practically administered by oral, rectal, or transdermal routes

Practical Considerations

- Cost
- Availability in local pharmacies
- Amount of opioid needed
- Route of administration
- Patient preference

6-Step Approach to Opioid Conversion[2–5]

See Appendix 15 for an opioid conversion table and Appendix 18 for a list of opioid conversion calculators.

1. **Globally assess** the patient to determine if the uncontrolled pain is secondary to worsening of disease or development of a new type of pain.
   - Tip: Treat the patient, *not* the table.
   - Tip: Use only one conversion table.
   - Tip: Start conservatively; then titrate to effect.

2. **Determine the *total* daily usage of the current opioid.** This should include all long-acting and breakthrough opioid doses.
   - Tip: Calculate doses based on *24-hour usage*.
   - Tip: Don't forget rescue doses.
   - The American Pain Society's *Principles of Analgesic Use in the Treatment of Acute Pain and Cancer Pain*[5] indicates that dose changes for patients on high doses of opioids may best be accomplished in stages by first implementing a partial conversion to minimize the risks of serious miscalculation (withdrawal, severe pain, overdose).
     - For example, a patient being changed from an intravenous (IV) to an oral opioid preparation might have his/her infu-

sion decreased by 50%, with the remaining 50% of the opioid requirement provided by an oral formulation.

* Reassessment of this strategy can be made after 24 hours.

3. **Decide which new opioid analgesic will be used** and consult the established conversion tables to arrive at the proper dose of the new opioid, recognizing the limitations of the data.

 ■ Remember that the doses listed are only estimates and can vary; the optimal dose for any individual patient is always determined by careful titration and appropriate monitoring.

 ■ Comparisons between intramuscular (IM) and IV doses of different opioids are not always clear. It is recommended that IV doses be based on two assumptions[5]:

 * Half the IV dose will give the same peak effect as a single IM dose.

 * IV and IM total doses should be equal when calculating the 24-hour requirements as IM doses are eventually fully absorbed.

 ■ If switching to any opioid other than methadone or fentanyl, decrease the dose by 25% to 50%.

 ■ If switching to methadone, reduce the dose by 75% to 90%.

 ■ If switching to transdermal fentanyl, do not reduce the dose.

4. **Opioid rotation** for patients on high doses is not straightforward and **may require consultation** and possibly hospitalization, especially when switching to methadone.

5. **Individualize the dose** based on information gathered in Step 1, and ensure adequate access to breakthrough medication.

 ■ Take the half-life of opioids into consideration when changing patients to different opioids.

 * Estimates of doses will vary widely depending on the half-life of the initial and replacement opioid, sometimes resulting in doses several times as large as the original dose.

- When there is concern that inadequate treatment of severe pain during opioid conversion may result from underdosing due to safety concerns about overestimating the conversion dose, hospitalization during dose conversion may be appropriate.

6. **Follow up with the patient** and **continually reassess,** especially during the first 7 to 14 days, to fine-tune the total daily dose (long-acting plus short-acting) and increase (or decrease) the around-the-clock long-acting dose accordingly.
   - Tip: Know the medications you are using.
   - Tip: Get help.

Continuing Opioid Therapy with Current Regimen

- Continuation of opioid therapy is appropriate under the following circumstances:
  - **The patient is doing well** on the current analgesic regimen:
    - Satisfactory pain relief
    - Stable or improving function
    - Tolerable side effects
    - Compliance with the rules of therapy
  - The patient's therapy is *not* optimal, but working with the **current opioid is appropriate.**
- If the patient's regimen is **suboptimal,** the modifications in the following table should be considered.

If the modifications to the current regimen suggested in this table do not solve the problem, then alternatives should be pursued (opioid rotation or exit strategy; see pages 33, 41).

Adjusting Current Opioid: Common Scenarios

Problem	Solution
Fixed doses only (e.g., oxycodone ER 40 mg q12h)	
Side effects (with good pain relief)	Decrease dose
Inadequate pain relief (but *no significant side effects*)	Increase dose
	Add nonpharmacologic therapy (see Appendix 12)
Inadequate pain relief (*with side effects*)	Add a nonopioid analgesic* (see Appendix 12)
	Lower opioid dose
	If possible, treat specific side effect
	Add nonpharmacologic therapy (see Appendix 12)
	Rotate to another opioid (see page 33)
Breakthrough pain in a compliant patient	Add a short-acting opioid for breakthrough pain (see page 23 and Appendix 13)
Compliance problems	Reinforce treatment agreement (see Appendix 17)
	Re-triage patient (see page 19)
As-needed doses only (e.g., hydrocodone/acetaminophen 1–2 tabs tid prn)	
Side effects (with good pain relief)	Decrease dose
Inadequate pain relief (but *no significant side effects*)	Increase dose, but do not exceed maximum recommended amount
	Add long-acting opioid if improving patient convenience would be useful (see page 23 and Appendix 13)
	Add nonpharmacologic therapy (see Appendix 12)

(continued)

Problem	Solution
Inadequate pain relief (*with side effects*)	Add a nonopioid analgesic* (see Appendix 12)
	Lower opioid dose
	If possible, treat specific side effect (see page 29)
	Add nonpharmacologic therapy (see Appendix 12)
Requirement for frequent prn doses is inconvenient (but *no significant side effects*)	Add a long-acting opioid in fixed doses (see page 23 and Appendix 13)
Fixed background opioid and prn opioid	
Compliance problems	Reinforce treatment agreement (see Appendix 17)
	Re-triage patient (see page 19)
	Consider replacing prn opioid with fixed-dose long-acting opioid
Side effects occur after prn doses (with good pain relief)	Decrease dose of prn medication
Side effects all the time	Decrease background dose
Inadequate pain relief around the clock (but *no significant side effects*)	Increase background dose
prn doses do not adequately relieve breakthrough pain (but *no significant side effects*)	Increase dose of prn medication
Inadequate pain relief (*with side effects*)	Add a nonopioid analgesic* (see Appendix 12)
	Lower opioid dose
	If possible, treat specific side effect (see page 29)
	Add nonpharmacologic therapy (see Appendix 12)

(continued)

Problem	Solution
Requirement for frequent prn doses is inconvenient (but *no significant side effects*)	Increase background dose
Compliance problems	Reinforce opioid agreement (see Appendix 17)
	Re-triage patient (see page 19)
	Consider eliminating prn medication

*Note: Potential presence of nonopioid analgesics in combination products; see Appendix 12.

Exit Strategy: Tapering/ Discontinuation

■ Review exit strategy[6] (see Appendix 16).

■ Document lack of pain reduction and/or lack of functional improvement.

■ Reinforce with patient that exit criteria were specified in the patient medication agreement.

■ Distinguish between abandoning opioid therapy, abandoning pain management, and abandoning patient.

■ Taper off opioid therapy, with or without specialty assistance.

■ Continue nonopioid pain management and general medical care.

Glossary

Abuse   The use of a substance to modify or control mood or state of mind in a manner that is illegal or harmful to oneself or others. Examples of the potential consequences of harmful use include accidents or injuries, blackouts, legal problems, and sexual behaviors that potentially increase the risk of human immunodeficiency virus infection.

Addiction   A primary, chronic, neurobiologic disease, with genetic, psychosocial, and environmental factors influencing its development and manifestations. Characterized by behaviors that include one or more of the following: impaired control over drug use, compulsive use, craving, and continued use despite harm.

Diversion   Redirecting the supply of legally obtainable medications into illegal channels, or the obtaining of a controlled substance by an illegal method.

Misuse   The use of a substance in a manner not consistent with legal or medical guidelines (such as altering dosing or sharing medicines), which has harmful or potentially harmful consequences. Misuse can be intentional or unintentional. *Does not refer to use for mind-altering purposes.*

Physical dependence   A state of adaptation that is manifested by a withdrawal syndrome that can be produced by abrupt cessation, rapid dose reduction, or administration of an antagonist.

Pseudoaddiction   Abuse-like behaviors that may develop in response to the undertreatment of pain. Examples include becoming focused on obtaining medications, "clock watching," and other "drug-seeking" behaviors.

Psychoactive substance use   The use of a psychoactive drug in a socially accepted or medically sanctioned manner to modify or control mood or state of mind, in the absence of harmful consequences or a pattern of use likely to lead to harmful consequences. Examples include having a drink with a friend, or taking an antianxiety agent for an acute anxiety state in accordance with a physician's prescription.

Tolerance   Loss of a drug's effects over time or the need to increase the dose to maintain the effect.

Withdrawal   A syndrome that occurs due to the cessation or reduction of prolonged use of a drug. Acute opioid withdrawal is characterized by dysphoria, nausea or vomiting, muscle aches, lacrimation, rhinorrhea, pupillary dilation, diarrhea, yawning, fever, or insomnia.

Appendix 1

Instructions for Office Staff: Setting Up a System for Safe Opioid Prescribing

- Inform your patients about their legal responsibilities with respect to controlled substances.
  - Some offices choose to put up a sign, such as the one in Appendix 3, which is based on Massachusetts law.
  - Decide whether or not this sign will state your office's policy about calling the police.
  - Some offices choose to incorporate this information in patient education materials that are provided to patients receiving controlled substances.
- Flag the charts of all patients on opioid therapy in a private and nonstigmatizing manner (e.g., with a colored sticker). Charts can be flagged for each patient visit.
- Use only tamper- and copy-proof prescription pads; serialized pads are even better.
- Keep prescription pads in a secure location.
- For electronic medical records systems: Use software that includes automatic dosing safeguards and that also alerts the PCP when there are frequent opioid prescriptions for an individual patient.

Urine Toxicology

- Develop an arrangement with a provider for quantitative urine medication monitoring **appropriate to opioid therapy.** Although accepted standards are not yet available, consider the following guidelines:
  - The laboratory assay should be as specific as possible (i.e., the fewest false-positive drug identifications).

- The assay should have the lowest limit of quantification possible, to avoid false-negative results (i.e., the drug was present but not detected).
- The test **must** be able to distinguish between one prescribed opioid and another.
- The test should also detect other prescribed controlled medications (e.g., benzodiazepines), illicit drugs, and alcohol.
- The laboratory should offer consultation with a clinical pathologist who is experienced in urine medication monitoring when questions arise; questions are inevitable.

Patient Visits

- Have the patient provide a **urine specimen** before seeing the PCP. Advise patients to refrain from urinating for as long as possible before the visit, and to arrive early for these procedures.
- Schedule the patient for necessary **blood tests,** if endocrine laboratory tests have not been obtained or are older than 12 months.
- Have the patient complete a **mental health screening tool** (see Appendix 9), if not previously completed, or if screen is older than 12 months.
- Set up examination room as follows:
  - To ensure that the required tools are readily available in each room where the clinician will be evaluating patients, **set up a file organized by type of visit** (e.g., initial patient assessment, opioid trial initiation, follow-up visit, etc.). Insert copies of the tools listed in Appendix 4 to create a packet that can be quickly removed and added to the patient's chart.

■ **Prepare patient's chart:** Make sure that it includes information appropriate to the type of patient visit, as follows:

	Initial Patient Assessment Visit	Follow-Up Visits for Patients on Opioid Therapy
Endocrine laboratory test results		X
Exit strategy tool (see Appendix 16)		X
Follow-up visit form (see Appendix 14)		X
Initial patient evaluation guide (see Appendix 6)	X	
Medication flow chart (see Appendix 2)	X	X
Mental health screening tool (completed by patient; see Appendix 9)	X	X
Patient medication agreement (signed by patient; see Appendix 17)	X	
Prescription monitoring report (most recent copy; in states where the report is available)		X
Triage tool (see page 19)	X	
Urine medication monitoring results (and all past results)		X

Appendix 2

Medication Flow Chart

Patient name _____

Patient ID _____

Allergies _____

Date of Prescription	Medication Name (brand/generic)	Strength (e.g., 25 mg)	Directions (e.g., 1–2 tabs tid pm)	# of Dosage Units Dispensed (e.g., 90)	Days' Supply (e.g., 30 days)	# of Refills	Date Due for New Prescription	Date(s) Prescription Refilled	Date and Reason for Discontinuation of Medication

Appendix 3

Controlled Substances Policy Notice

It is a felony under state* law, punishable by fine and imprisonment, to:

- Obtain (or attempt to obtain) possession of a controlled substance by means of forgery, fraud, or deception.
- Forge or falsify a prescription, or not disclose a material fact, in order to obtain a controlled substance from a practitioner.

It is our policy to report this crime to the police.

*Check with your local authorities for specific details.

Appendix 4

**Tools for the Primary Care Physician
to Use during Office Visits**

Type of Visit	Tool
Initial patient assessment	Initial evaluation guide (see Appendix 6)
	SOAPP® (see Appendix 7)
	Triage guide (see page 19)
	Mental health screening tool (see Appendix 9)
	Urine medication monitoring (see Appendix 10)
Opioid trial initiation	Patient medication agreement (see Appendix 17)
	Medication table (see Appendix 13)
Follow-up visit	Follow-up visit form (see Appendix 14)
	COMM™ (see Appendix 8)
	Medication flow chart (see Appendix 2)
	Urine medication monitoring (see Appendix 10)
	Prescription monitoring program report (see page 13)
	Endocrine laboratory tests (annually) (see Appendix 10)
Conversion to long-acting opioid	Conversion/rotation tool (see Appendix 15)
Opioid rotation	Conversion/rotation tool (see Appendix 15)
Taper opioid therapy	Exit strategy for discontinuing opioid therapy (see Appendix 16)

Appendix 5

Recognizing Prescription Opioid Abusers[6,7]

General Indicators

- Deteriorating personal appearance and hygiene
- Appears intoxicated
- Appears sedated or confused (e.g., slurred speech, unresponsive)
- Expresses worries about addiction
- Exhibits lack of interest in rehabilitation or self-management
- Abuses alcohol or uses illicit drugs
- Arrested by police
- Victim of abuse
- Increasingly negative moods
- Mood swings appear to occur at similar times of the day
- Overly reactive to admonishments or compliments
- Increasingly complains about co-workers, family, or friends
- Worsened relationships with family
- Family or significant others express concern over patient's use of analgesics
- Deliberately avoids co-workers and supervisors, especially those who have been trained to spot abusers
- Careless; makes frequent mistakes and shows poor judgment
- Involvement in car or other accident (3.6 times more likely to have an accident at work and 9 times more likely to have a domestic or car accident)
- Frequent and recurring financial problems

Work-Related Indicators

- Frequently late to work
- Requests early dismissal or time off (2.2 times more often)

- Frequently uses sick leave (3 times more often)
- Frequently files worker compensation claims (5 times more likely)

Medication-Related Indicators

- Purposeful over-sedation
- Uses pain medication in response to stress
- Uses analgesics prn when prescription is for time-contingent use
- Uses more analgesic than prescribed
- Requests frequent early renewals or runs out of medications early
- Reports lost or stolen prescriptions
- Attempts to obtain prescriptions from other doctors
- Hoards or stockpiles medication
- Buys medication on the street
- Changes route of administration
- Insists on certain medications by name
- Expresses a strong preference for a specific type of analgesic or a specific route of administration
- Expresses concern about future availability of controlled substance
- Misrepresents analgesic prescription or use
- Indicates he/she "must have" analgesic
- Predominant issue of office visit is discussion of analgesic medication
- Reports minimal or inadequate relief from opioid analgesic
- Difficulty adhering to medication agreement

Notes:

- Some of these behaviors can be normal.
- None of these behaviors is diagnostic.
- Take a therapeutic approach with your patient.
- Set limits.

Appendix 6

Initial Evaluation Guide

History of Present Illness (Pain)

Pain Assessment: What and How

- As with any other clinical condition, a detailed general history and physical examination is appropriate in every case.
- Several pain assessment tools are available (see Appendices 14 and 18).
- These tools provide a systematic process for characterizing the pain, noting aspects of previous treatment, and documenting the effect of pain on other dimensions of the patient's life.
- Sample questions:
  - What is the type of pain?
  - Where is it located?
  - How severe is it?
  - What makes it worse?
  - What makes it better?
  - What side effects were experienced with previous pain relief therapies?
  - What is the effect on the patient's mood or energy?
  - Use a pain scale like the one below to gauge pain levels:
    - What was the patient's pain level on average during the past week?
    - What was the patient's worst pain level during the past week?
    - What was the patient's least pain level during the past week?

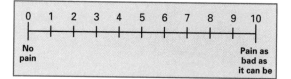

- How much has pain affected your life?
- Is the amount of pain relief you are now obtaining from your current pain reliever(s) enough to make a real difference? (yes or no)
- Previous pain treatments?
- Previous experience with opioid therapy?
  - Effectiveness of opioid therapy on pain and function?
  - Compliance?
  - Subjective experience with opioid therapy (e.g., euphoria)?
  - Use of opioids for nonprescribed purposes (e.g., insomnia, "stress," mood)?

History and Physical Examination: Features Relevant to Substance Abuse

History

Past Medical History
- Illnesses relevant to effects or metabolism of opioid therapy (e.g., respiratory, hepatic, renal disease)
- Medical illnesses suggestive of substance abuse:
  - Hepatitis
  - Human immunodeficiency virus
  - Tuberculosis
  - Cellulitis
  - Sexually transmitted diseases
- Elevated liver function tests
- Trauma, burns

Psychiatric History
- Current or past mental illness (see Appendix 9 for Mental Health Screening Tool)

Substance Abuse History
- History of substance abuse, including illicit or prescription:
  - None

- Past, in remission
- Current
- Routes
- Alcohol:
  - None
  - Past
  - Current
- Tobacco:
  - None
  - Past
  - Current

Social History
- Arrests
- Motor vehicle accidents; driving under the influence
- Domestic violence
- Fires
- Contact with substance abusers

Family History
- Substance abuse
- Family support
- Psychiatric

Physical Examination

Skin
- Abscesses, cellulitis, and tissue necrosis—signs of drug use
- Parallel needle marks; hyperpigmentation overlying a vein
- Palpably sclerotic veins
- Trauma to skin (e.g., abrasions, lacerations, cigarette burns)

Head and Neck
- Perforation of nasal septum, especially for those using stimulants
- Poor dentition (especially opioid and stimulant abusers)

Chest
- Cardiac disease (all types of drug users)

- Pulmonary disease due to smoking drugs (although most drug abusers are also heavy tobacco users)
- Pulmonary diseases due to suppression of respiration and cough reflex

Abdomen
- Hepatomegaly and liver tenderness due to hepatitis
- Splenomegaly in parenteral drug users

Lymphatic System
- Adenopathy, especially in groin and axillae (common injection sites for IV drug users)

Nervous System
- Peripheral neuropathies
  - Sometimes secondary to tissue necrosis from injection
  - Also seen in alcohol and drug abusers

Additional Laboratory Tests (see Appendix 10)
- Urine medication monitoring
- Endocrine tests
- Other blood tests as appropriate

Appendix 7

Screener and Opioid Assessment for Patients with Pain (SOAPP®)

■ SOAPP® Version 1.0, 24-Item

SOAPP Question	Rate on Scale of 0–4 (0 = never; 4 = usually, or frequently)
1. How often do you feel that your pain is "out of control?"	
2. How often do you have mood swings?	
3. How often do you do things that you later regret?	
4. How often has your family been supportive and encouraging?	
5. How often have others told you that you have a bad temper?	
6. Compared with other people, how often have you been in a car accident?	
7. How often do you smoke a cigarette within an hour after you wake up?	
8. How often have you felt a need for higher doses of medication to treat your pain?	
9. How often do you take more medication than you are supposed to?	
10. How often have any of your family members, including parents and grandparents, had a problem with alcohol or drugs?	
11. How often have any of your close friends had a problem with alcohol or drugs?	
	(continued)

■ SOAPP® Version 1.0, 24-Item

SOAPP Question	Rate on Scale of 0–4 (0 = never; 4 = usually, or frequently)
12. How often have others suggested that you have a drug or alcohol problem?	
13. How often have you attended an AA or NA meeting?	
14. How often have you had a problem getting along with the doctors who prescribed your medicines?	
15. How often have you taken medication other than the way that it was prescribed?	
16. How often have you been seen by a psychiatrist or a mental health counselor?	
17. How often have you been treated for an alcohol or drug problem?	
18. How often have your medications been lost or stolen?	
19. How often have others expressed concern over your use of medication?	
20. How often have you felt a craving for medication?	
21. How often has more than one doctor prescribed pain medication for you at the same time?	
22. How often have you been asked to give a urine screen for substance abuse?	
23. How often have you used illegal drugs (for example, marijuana, cocaine, etc.) in the past five years?	
24. How often, in your lifetime, have you had legal problems or been arrested?	
Total	

Please see *http://www.PainEDU.org* for more information about the SOAPP, including instructions and scoring. You may also view the tutorial at the site, or download the tool.

■ 14-Item SOAPP®

SOAPP Question	Rate on Scale of 0–4 (0 = never; 4 = usually, or frequently)
1. How often do you have mood swings?	
2. How often do you smoke a cigarette within an hour after you wake up?	
3. How often have any of your family members, including parents and grandparents, had a problem with alcohol or drugs?	
4. How often have any of your close friends had a problem with alcohol or drugs?	
5. How often have others suggested that you have a drug or alcohol problem?	
6. How often have you attended an AA or NA meeting?	
7. How often have you taken medication other than the way that it was prescribed?	
8. How often have you been treated for an alcohol or drug problem?	
9. How often have your medications been lost or stolen?	
10. How often have others expressed concern over your use of medication?	
11. How often have you felt a craving for medication?	
12. How often have you been asked to give a urine screen for substance abuse?	
13. How often have you used illegal drugs (for example, marijuana, cocaine, etc.) in the past five years?	

(continued)

■ 14-Item SOAPP®

SOAPP Question	Rate on Scale of 0–4 (0 = never; 4 = usually, or frequently)
14. How often, in your lifetime, have you had legal problems or been arrested?	
Total	

Please see *http://www.PainEDU.org* for more information about the SOAPP, including instructions and scoring. You may also view the tutorial at the site, or download the tool.

■ 5-Item SOAPP® (SOAPP-SF)

SOAPP Question	Rate on Scale of 0–4 (0 = never; 4 = usually, or frequently)
1. How often do you have mood swings?	
2. How often do you smoke a cigarette within an hour after you wake up?	
3. How often have you taken medication other than in the way that it was prescribed?	
4. How often have you used illegal drugs (for example, marijuana, cocaine, etc.) in the past five years?	
5. How often, in your lifetime, have you had legal problems or been arrested?	
Total	

Please see *http://www.PainEDU.org* for more information about the SOAPP, including instructions and scoring. You may also view the tutorial at the site, or download the tool.

■ SOAPP®-R (Revised Version)

SOAPP Question	Rate on Scale of 0–4 (0 = never; 4 = usually, or frequently)
1. How often do you have mood swings?	
2. How often have you felt a need for higher doses of medication to treat your pain?	
3. How often have you felt impatient with your doctors?	
4. How often have you felt that things are just too overwhelming that you can't handle them?	
5. How often is there tension in the home?	
6. How often have you counted pain pills to see how many are remaining?	
7. How often have you been concerned that people will judge you for taking pain medication?	
8. How often do you feel bored?	
9. How often have you taken more pain medication than you were supposed to?	
10. How often have you worried about being left alone?	
11. How often have you felt a craving for medication?	
12. How often have others expressed concern over your use of medication?	
13. How often have any of your close friends had a problem with alcohol or drugs?	
14. How often have others told you that you had a bad temper?	
15. How often have you felt consumed by the need to get pain medication?	
	(continued)

■ SOAPP®-R (Revised Version)

SOAPP Question	Rate on Scale of 0–4 (0 = never; 4 = usually, or frequently)
16. How often have you run out of pain medication early?	
17. How often have others kept you from getting what you deserve?	
18. How often, in your lifetime, have you had legal problems or been arrested?	
19. How often have you attended an AA or NA meeting?	
20. How often have you been in an argument that was so out of control that someone got hurt?	
21. How often have you been sexually abused?	
22. How often have others suggested that you have a drug or alcohol problem?	
23. How often have you had to borrow pain medications from your family or friends?	
24. How often have you been treated for an alcohol or drug problem?	
Total	

Please see *http://www.PainEDU.org* for more information about the SOAPP, including instructions and scoring. You may also view the tutorial at the site, or download the tool. Abbreviations: AA = Alcoholics Anonymous; NA = Narcotics Anonymous. ©2010 Inflexxion, Inc. Permissions questions: *PainEDU@inflexxion.com*. The SOAPP® was developed with a grant from the National Institutes of Health and an educational grant from Endo Pharmaceuticals.

Suggested Readings

Butler SF, Budman SH, Fernandez K, Jamison RN. Validation of a screener and opioid assessment measure for patients with chronic pain. *Pain.* 2004;112:65–75.

Butler SF, Fernandez K, Benoit C, Budman SH, Jamison RN. Validation of the revised Screener and Opioid Assessment for Patients with Pain (SOAPP-R). *J Pain* 2008 Apr;9(4):360–72. Epub 2008 Jan 22.

Chou R, Fanciullo GJ, Fine PG, et al. Clinical guidelines for the use of chronic opioid therapy in chronic noncancer pain. *J Pain* 2009; 10(2):113–130.

Moore TM, Jones T, Browder JH, Daffron S, Passik SD. A comparison of common screening methods for predicting aberrant drug-related behavior among patients receiving opioids for chronic pain management. *Pain Med* 2009;10(8):1426–1433.

Appendix 8

Current Opioid Misuse Measure (COMM)®

COMM Question	Rate on Scale of 0–4 (0 = never; 4 = very often)
1. In the past 30 days, how often have you had trouble with thinking clearly or had memory problems?	
2. In the past 30 days, how often do people complain that you are not completing necessary tasks? (i.e., doing things that need to be done, such as going to class, work or appointments)	
3. In the past 30 days, how often have you had to go to someone other than your prescribing physician to get sufficient pain relief from medications? (i.e., another doctor, the Emergency Room, friends, street sources)	
4. In the past 30 days, how often have you taken your medications differently from how they are prescribed?	
5. In the past 30 days, how often have you seriously thought about hurting yourself?	
6. In the past 30 days, how much of your time was spent thinking about opioid medications (having enough, taking them, dosing schedule, etc.)?	
7. In the past 30 days, how often have you been in an argument?	
8. In the past 30 days, how often have you had trouble controlling your anger (e.g., road rage, screaming, etc.)?	
	(continued)

COMM Question	Rate on Scale of 0–4 (0 = never; 4 = very often)
9. In the past 30 days, how often have you needed to take pain medications belonging to someone else?	
10. In the past 30 days, how often have you been worried about how you're handling your medications?	
11. In the past 30 days, how often have others been worried about how you're handling your medications?	
12. In the past 30 days, how often have you had to make an emergency phone call or show up at the clinic without an appointment?	
13. In the past 30 days, how often have you gotten angry with people?	
14. In the past 30 days, how often have you had to take more of your medication than prescribed?	
15. In the past 30 days, how often have you borrowed pain medication from someone else?	
16. In the past 30 days, how often have you used your pain medicine for symptoms other than for pain (e.g., to help you sleep, improve your mood, or relieve stress)?	
17. In the past 30 days, how often have you had to visit the Emergency Room?	
Total	

Please see *http://www.PainEDU.org* for more information about the COMM, including instructions, scoring, or download the tool.

©2010 Inflexxion, Inc. Permissions questions: *PainEDU@inflexxion.com*. The Current Opioid Misuse Measure (COMM)® was developed with a grant from the National Institutes of Health and an educational grant from Endo Pharmaceuticals.

Suggested Reading

Butler SF, Budman SH, Fernandez KC, et al. Development and validation of the Current Opioid Misuse Measure. *Pain* 2007;130(1–2):144–156. Epub 2007 May 9.

Appendix 9

Mental Health Screening Tool

	All of the time	Most of the time	Some of the time	A little of the time	None of the time
1. During the past month, how much of the time were you a happy person?	5	4	3	2	1
2. How much of the time, during the past month, have you felt calm and peaceful?	5	4	3	2	1
3. How much of the time, during the past month, have you been a very nervous person?	1	2	3	4	5
4. How much of the time, during the past month, have you felt down-hearted and blue?	1	2	3	4	5

(continued)

Mental Health Screening Tool (Continued)

	All of the time	Most of the time	Some of the time	A little of the time	None of the time
5. How much of the time, during the past month, did you feel so down in the dumps that nothing could cheer you up?	1	2	3	4	5
				Sum of Answers _____	
				FINAL SCORE _____	

Scoring the Mental Health Screening Tool

1. Add up the points, and write the total at the bottom of the right-hand column ("Sum of Answers")
2. To get the **Final Score:**
    * Subtract 5 from the Sum of Answers. Divide by 20.
    * Multiply result by 100.
    * Calculate: (Sum of Answers – 5) / 20 = _____ × 100 = Final Score
3. A Final Score of less than 52 is clinically significant and should trigger a mental health referral to a practitioner who is experienced with chronic pain.

The Mental Health Inventory-5 (MHI-5), part of the Medical Outcomes Study, is reproduced here, in part, with permission from the RAND Corporation. Copyright© RAND Corporation. RAND's permission to reproduce the survey is not an endorsement of the products, services, or other uses in which the survey appears or is applied.

Suggested Reading

Veit CT, Ware JE, Jr. The structure of psychological distress and well-being in general populations. *J Consult Clin Psychol* 1983;51:730–742.

Appendix 10

Laboratory Tests

Urine Tests

Urine drug screening can play an important role in monitoring patients for aberrant drug-related behavior.[8]

- In most circumstances, periodic, randomized urine testing is recommended.
- Urine tests should be conducted to include screening for:
  - Cocaine
  - Heroin
  - Amphetamines
  - Marijuana
  - Prescription opioids
  - Benzodiazepines
  - Alcohol
- Unobserved urine collection may be acceptable.
- A number of aspects of the urine can indicate that it has been adulterated. Establish testing protocols with the urine toxicology testing provider.
- Develop a relationship with a urine drug-testing laboratory (see Appendix 1).
- **If any unexpected laboratory results are found:**
  - Consult with the laboratory about their significance.
  - Schedule an appointment with the patient to discuss results.
- A positive, supportive approach enhances both the patient's readiness to change and his/her opportunities for motivational enhancement therapy.
- Use results to strengthen the health care professional/patient relationship and to support positive behavior change.
  - Chart results and interpretation.

- Causes of false positives:
  - Some opioids are metabolized to other compounds and may confound results. Examples include:
    - Codeine, which is metabolized to morphine.
    - Hydrocodone, which is metabolized to hydromorphone.
  - As a result, primary care clinicians should not be alarmed if these opioids are found in the urine of patients being treated with codeine or hydrocodone.
  - Contact the laboratory directly if you have any questions about test results.
- Causes of false negatives:
  - The absence of a prescribed opioid in the urine can occur for technical reasons. This result alone does not indicate that the patient is not taking the medication.

Blood Tests

Routine screening for opioid-induced hypogonadism is indicated for all patients on long-term opioid therapy. Opioid-induced hypogonadism is a common complication of opioid therapy in both men and women, occurring in the majority of patients in some studies. With the rising use of opioids for chronic pain, patient monitoring is increasingly important in order to manage possible endocrine complications. Symptoms may be subtle, and may include fatigue, mood changes, decreased libido, loss of muscle mass, and osteoporosis.

Depending on clinical presentation, some of the following tests may be indicated.

Screening of Men
- Hormone evaluations*
  - Total testosterone
  - Sex hormone binding globulin (SHBG)
  - Luteinizing hormone (LH), with optional follicle-stimulating hormone (FSH)
  - Free testosterone
  - Prolactin

Screening of Women

- ■ Hormone evaluations*
  - ■ Total testosterone
  - ■ SHBG
  - ■ LH
    - • May be low from opioids
  - ■ FSH
    - • Should be elevated in menopause but may be low from opioids
  - ■ Free testosterone
  - ■ Prolactin
  - ■ Dehydroepiandrosterone sulfate
  - ■ Free cortisol (serum)
    - • Often low in women on opioids

Premenopausal women (not on oral or transdermal contraceptives)†

- ■ If patient is not having menstrual cycles, it could be a sign of opioid effect or pregnancy.
  - ■ Perform pregnancy test (if suspected).

Women on hormonal contraceptives or estrogen therapy‡

- ■ SHBG levels may be elevated from oral estrogen administration.
- ■ LH/FSH levels may additionally be lowered from oral or transdermal estrogen therapy.
- ■ Free testosterone levels may be even lower than in postmenopausal women who are not on estrogen therapy or estrogen/progestin therapy, or premenopausal women not on oral or transdermal contraceptives.

Note: Testosterone therapy is not yet established for women; there are no specific recommendations for monitoring therapy. Premenopausal women who have stopped menstruating may want to go on oral contraceptives concurrently with opioids, in order to protect against irregular ovulations and unwanted pregnancy.

*Hormone samples are preferably obtained between 7 AM and noon.
†If women are having menstrual cycles, obtain sample between days 3 and 8.

‡Samples can be obtained at any time in ovulation cycle, preferably in morning for standardization.

Suggested Readings

Daniell HW, Lentz R, Mazer NA. Open-label pilot study of testosterone patch therapy in men with opioid-induced androgen deficiency. *J Pain* 2006;7:200–10.

Daniell HW. DHEAS deficiency during consumption of sustained-action prescribed opioids: evidence for opioid-induced inhibition of adrenal androgen production. *J Pain* 2006;7:901–7.

Bhasin S, Cunningham GR, Hayes FJ, et al. Testosterone therapy in adult men with androgen deficiency syndromes: an Endocrine Society Clinical Practice Guideline. *J Clin Endocrinol Metab* 2006;91:1995–2010. Erratum in: *J Clin Endocrinol Metab* 2006;91:2688.

Appendix 11

Screening and Brief Intervention in the Primary Care Office

PCPs have an opportunity to identify early signs of substance abuse by:

- Conducting screening for substance abuse:
  - Assess the patient for signs of emerging substance abuse (see Appendices 5 and 14)
  - Screen the patient by asking the following questions:
    - "In the past year, have you ever used alcohol, other drugs, or your prescription medication more than you meant to?"[9]
    - "Have you felt that you wanted to (or needed to) cut down on your use of prescription pain medication in the past year?"[9]

A "yes" response, or other positive indicators, may signify the possibility of emerging substance abuse. When clinical judgment supports this possibility, the PCP should state something to the patient that is similar to the following script (adapted to the patient's specific situation):

- "I'm concerned that your use of _____ is more than is medically safe. I am especially concerned that you might be developing a problem with your use of the medication. Others who have used this medication the way you are using it have had serious medical problems or, in some cases, have even stopped breathing. If not already a problem, you may begin to have one or more of the following difficulties:
  - Mood swings that affect your relationships with family and friends, at work or at school
  - Worsening of your personal appearance and hygiene, and increasing carelessness, which can cause problems at work or school, as well as at home
  - Car accidents or accidents at home."

For patients who have been unable to remain compliant with medications or other substances, despite clear feedback:

■ "I recommend that we begin to gradually withdraw your opioid pain medication. We will accomplish this by reducing the dose of _____, which you are currently taking, by half every _____ day(s) until you are completely off the medication. In its place, I recommend that we begin treating your pain with _____. This is a nonnarcotic way of treating you that I believe will be effective and has no risk of addiction."

For patients who may be compliant, but have signs of a potential emerging addiction:

■ "I will arrange for you to see _____, an addiction specialist I trust, who will help evaluate your situation and provide recommendations for treatment. I also recommend that you join a support group for people like yourself who have problems with prescription medications or other substances. The nearest one to your home is located at this address:_____, and meetings are held every _____ at _____ o'clock.

I'm going to continue to work with you through this process and have arranged a follow-up appointment to see you again in 2 weeks. I don't want you to be discouraged. Change is difficult, but I know you can do this."

■ If referring the patient, ask the addiction specialist to provide summary reports on the patient's progress.

■ Rescreen the patient annually for substance abuse.

Suggested Reading

Center for Substance Abuse Treatment. *Substance Abuse Treatment for Persons With Co-Occurring Disorders.* Treatment Improvement Protocol (TIP) Series 42. DHHS Publication No. (SMA) 05-3922. Rockville, MD: Substance Abuse and Mental Health Services Administration, 2005. *http://www.ncbi. nlm.nih.gov/bookshelf/br.fcgi?book=hssamhsatip&part=A74073#A74073.*

Appendix 12

**Nonpharmacologic and Nonopioid
Analgesic Treatment of Chronic Pain**

- In most cases, the treatment of pain should begin with non-pharmacologic measures, along with, or without, pharmacotherapy:
  - Ice
  - Heat
  - Corsets
  - Exercise
  - Rehabilitation
  - Cognitive-behavioral therapy
- If these measures are ineffective, a variety of common nonopioid analgesic medications (such as those in the following tables) are also available. Potential side effects are noted.

Nonopioid Analgesics

Drug	Potential Side Effects
Acetaminophen	Liver failure (rare, and most likely with overdose or history of alcohol abuse)
Aspirin	Abdominal pain, bleeding, edema, mental status change, nausea/vomiting, pruritus/rash
Nonselective NSAIDs	Abdominal pain, bleeding, congestive heart failure, constipation, edema, headache, hypertension, nausea/vomiting, pruritus/rash
COX-2–selective NSAIDs	Abdominal pain, congestive heart failure, edema, headache, hypertension, nausea/vomiting, pruritus/rash, cardiovascular thrombosis

NSAIDs = nonsteroidal anti-inflammatory drugs.

Adjuvant Analgesics

Medication	Usual Starting Dose and Interval	Common Dosage Range
Antidepressants		
Amitriptyline	25 mg po hs (10 mg in frail, elderly)	50–150 mg po hs
Desipramine	25 mg po hs (10 mg in frail, elderly)	50–200 mg po hs
Nortriptyline	25 mg po hs (10 mg in frail, elderly)	50–150 mg po hs
Anticonvulsants		
Carbamazepine	100 mg po bid	200 mg po bid-qid
Clonazepam	0.25–0.5 mg po tid	0.5–1.0 mg po tid
Duloxetine	60 mg/day po	120 mg/day
Gabapentin	100 mg po tid; increase by 100 mg tid q3days	300–3600 mg/day in 3 divided doses
Pregabalin (for neuropathic pain; diabetic peripheral neuropathy)	100 mg po tid; start 50 mg tid; increase to 300 mg/ day over 7 days	Max: 300 mg/day
Valproic acid/ Divalproex	125 mg po tid	500–1000 mg po tid
Anxiolytics – Azapirones		
Buspirone	5 mg po tid	Max: 60 mg/day
Venlafaxine	75 mg bid or tid (immediate-release tablets) or qd (extended-release tablet) Increase of up to 75 mg/ day every few days	Max: 225 mg/day Some patients may benefit from higher doses. Monitor blood pressure and lipids.

(*continued*)

Medication	Usual Starting Dose and Interval	Common Dosage Range
Anxiolytics – Benzodiazepines (Note: All benzodiazepines cause additive sedation with opioids)		
Alprazolam	0.25–0.5 mg po qd-tid	Minimum effective dose
Chlordiazepoxide	10–25 mg po qd-tid	Minimum effective dose
Diazepam	5–10 mg po qd-bid	Minimum effective dose
Lorazepam	0.5–2 mg po qd-tid	Minimum effective dose
Midazolam	Doses vary depending on individual patient needs	
Corticosteroids		
Dexamethasone or methylpred-nisolone	Dexamethasone 40–100 mg IV or equivalent as loading doses or q6h for first 24–72 h (if indications are acute spinal cord compression, increased ICP)	Dexamethasone 10–20 mg IV q6h or methylpred-nisolone 40–80 mg IV q6h
	Dexamethasone 4–8 mg po q8–12h	Minimum effective dose
	Prednisone 20–40 mg po q8–12h (if indications are nerve compression, visceral distension, increased ICP, soft tissue infiltration)	
	Dexamethasone 4–12 mg/day	
	Prednisone 5–10 mg tid (if indications are alleviation of nausea, anorexia, pain in palliative care)	

(continued)

Medication	Usual Starting Dose and Interval	Common Dosage Range
Miscellaneous Adjuvant Analgesic Agents		
Baclofen	5–10 mg po tid-qid	Max: 80–120 mg/day (oral)
		Intrathecal: 300–800 mcg/day
Clonidine	30 pg/hr (epidural)	Doses > 40 mcg/hr not well studied
Mexiletene	150–300 mg po tid	150–300 mg po tid
Octreotide	50–100 mcg SC bid-tid	Varies
Pamidronate	90 mg IV q4wks	90 mg IV q4wks proven effective
Radiopharmaceuticals		
Strontium-89 Chloride	148 MBq, 4 mCi IV q3mos	148 MBq, 4 mCi q3mos
Samarium Sm 153 Lexidronam	1.0 mCi/kg IV	148 MBq, 4 mCi q3mos
Psychostimulants		
Dextroamphetamine	2.5–5.0 mg po qd or bid; last dose before 2 PM	5–20 mg in divided doses; last dose before 2 PM
Methylphenidate	2.5–5 mg po qd or bid; last dose before 2 PM	5–20 mg in divided doses; last dose before 2 PM
Modafinil	200 mg po qd	200 mg qd; occasionally patients may benefit from increasing to 400 mg qd
Topical Analgesics		
Capsaicin	0.025, 0.075% cream tid-qid	As directed

(*continued*)

Medication	Usual Starting Dose and Interval	Common Dosage Range
Diclofenac epolamine	1.3% topical patch; 1 patch bid	Minimum effective dose
Lidocaine	5% patch	Up to 12/hr/day; maximum 3 patches at a time
Lidocaine/ prilocaine topical	2.5%/2.5%	2.5 g on 20–25 cm of skin for patients older than age 2 yrs. Minimum effective dose

bid = twice daily; hs = at bedtime; ICP = intracranial pressure; IV = intravenous; MBq = megabecquerel; mCi = millicurie; po = by mouth; q = every; qd = daily; qid = 4 times a day; SC = subcutaneous; tid = 3 times a day.

Appendix 13

Dosing of Opioid Analgesics[10–12]

Table begins on page 88.

Table begins on page 88.

Drug	Recommended Starting Dose/Frequency (Adults >50 kg)		Recommended Starting Dose/Frequency (Child/Adults <50 kg)		Duration (Hours)	Comments
	Oral	Parenteral	Oral	Parenteral		
Codeine phosphate/sulfate	15–60 mg/q3–6h	IM/SC: 15–60 mg/q4–6h	0.5–1.0 mg/kg q4–6h	Not recommended	4–6	May be used for treatment of mild to moderate pain in conjunction with acetaminophen (analgesic and antitussive properties). Available as a combination with acetaminophen.
Fentanyl citrate IV, TD, B, TM	100–200 mcg (not to exceed 4 doses/day)	TD: 50 mcg/hr/72 hrs IV: 0.5–1.0 mcg/kg/dose	—	IV: 1–2 mcg/kg (as bolus) IV: 1–5 mcg/kg/hr (as continuous infusion)	IV: 0.5–1.0 TD: 72 B/TM: 2–4	IV use in institutional settings. May cause life-threatening hypoventilation in opioid-nontolerant patients. Generally, only indicated for cancer pain in opioid-tolerant patients with malignancies. Should be kept out of reach of children and discarded properly.

Drug					Half-life (h)	Comments
Hydrocodone HCL	2.5–10 mg q3–6h	—	0.2 mg/kg q3–6h	—	4–8	Concomitant use with moderate and strong CYP3A4 inhibitors may cause fatal respiratory depression. Available as a combination medication with acetaminophen, aspirin, or ibuprofen.
Hydromorphone HCL*	2–4 mg q3–6h	SC: 1–2 mg IM: 1–2 mg q3–4h	0.06 mg/kg q3–4h	IM: 0.015 mg/kg q3–4h	4–5	Available in a more concentrated injectable solution (HP), intended for use only in opioid-tolerant patients.
Levorphanol tartrate	2–4 mg/kg q6–8h	SC: 2–4 mg q6–8h	0.04 mg/kg q6–8h	SC: 0.02mg/kg q6–8h	6–8	The long half-life of the drug may increase the potential for drug accumulation and opioid-related adverse effects.
Meperidine HCL	50–150 mg q3–4h	SC: 100 mg IM: 100 mg	1.1–1.8 mg/kg q3–4h	SC/IM: 0.75 mg/kg q3–4h	2–4	Generally not recommended for general use due to its metabolite, normeperidine, which may accumulate and cause CNS effects, such as seizures.

(continued)

| Drug | Recommended Starting Dose/Frequency (Adults >50 kg) | | Recommended Starting Dose/Frequency (Child/Adults <50 kg) | | Duration (Hours) | Comments |
	Oral	Parenteral	Oral	Parenteral		
Methadone	5–10 mg q6–8h	SC: 10 mg IM: 10 mg q6–8h	0.2 mg/kg q6–8h	SC/IM: 0.1 mg/kg q6–8h	4–6	Higher level of potency when used chronically. Specialty consultation is advised when converting patients to methadone. Wait 1 week between dose increases. See Public Health Advisory.[†]
Morphine sulfate	IR: 15–30 mg q3–4h prn	SC: 10 mg IM: 10 mg IV: 2–4 mg q3–4h	0.3 mg/kg q4–6h	SC/IM: 0.1 mg/kg q4–8h	3–6	Once the daily morphine requirement is established, conversion to an extended or sustained-release formulation can be considered. Dosing should be equivalent to the patient's *daily* morphine requirement.

| Morphine sulfate/ naltrexone HCL[‡] (extended release) | 20 mg/0.8 mg in either single dose q24h or 50% divided dose q12h | — | Not recom- mended | Initially start at the lowest dose. Titrate and increase to qd or bid dosing. **Conversion from other Oral Morphine:** Give 50% of daily oral morphine dose q12h or give 100% oral morphine dose q24h. Do not give more frequently than q12h. **Conversion from Parenteral Morphine:** Oral morphine 3 times the daily parenteral morphine dose may be sufficient in chronic use settings. **Conversion from Other Parenteral or Oral Opioids:** Initial: Give 50% of estimated daily morphine demand and supplement with immediate-release morphine. Individualize dose in all patients. |

3–6

(continued)

Drug	Recommended Starting Dose/Frequency (Adults >50 kg)		Recommended Starting Dose/Frequency (Child/Adults <50 kg)		Duration (Hours)	Comments
	Oral	Parenteral	Oral	Parenteral		
Oxycodone	10 mg q12h	—	0.2mg/kg q3–4h	—	3–6	Available as a combination medication with acetaminophen, aspirin, or ibuprofen. (Roxicodone was withdrawn from the U.S. market in 2009.)
Oxymorphone HCL	IR: 10–20 mg q4–6h ER: 5–10 mg q12h	—	Not recommended	—	3–6	IR formulation indicated for the relief of moderate to severe acute pain where the use of an opioid is appropriate. ER formulation indicated for the relief of moderate to severe pain in patients requiring continuous, around-the-clock opioid treatment for an extended period of time.

Propoxyphene HCL	65–100 mg q4h	—	Not recommended	4–6	Weak analgesic and not recommended as first-line analgesic. Available as combination medication with acetaminophen, aspirin, and aspirin and caffeine.
Tramadol	IR: 50–100 mg q4–6h ER: 100 mg q24h	—	Not recommended	IR: 4–6 ER: 24	A centrally acting synthetic opioid analgesic. Although its mode of action is not completely understood, from animal tests, at least two complementary mechanisms appear applicable: binding of parent and M1 metabolite to μ-opioid receptors and weak inhibition of reuptake of norepinephrine and serotonin.

B = buccal; ER = extended-release; IM = intramuscular; IR = immediate release; IV = intravenous; prn = as needed; SC = subcutaneous; TD = transdermal; TM = transmucosal.

*U.S. Food and Drug Administration (FDA) approval of extended-release formulation available mid-2010.

†The FDA has received reports of death and life-threatening side effects in patients taking methadone. These deaths and life-threatening side effects have occurred in patients newly starting methadone for pain control and in patients who have switched to methadone after being treated for pain

with other strong narcotic pain relievers. Methadone can cause slow or shallow breathing and dangerous changes in heart beat that may not be felt by the patient. Prescribing methadone is complex. Methadone should only be prescribed for patients with moderate to severe pain when their pain is not improved with other nonnarcotic pain relievers. Pain relief from a dose of methadone lasts approximately 4 to 8 hours. However, methadone stays in the body much longer—from 8 to 59 hours after it is taken. As a result, patients may feel the need for more pain relief before methadone is gone from the body. Methadone may build up in the body to a toxic level if it is taken too often, or if it is taken with certain other medicines or supplements. **To prevent serious complications from methadone, health care professionals who prescribe methadone should read and carefully follow the methadone prescribing information.**

FDA is issuing this public health advisory to alert patients and their caregivers and health care professionals to the following important safety information: **1) Patients should take methadone exactly as prescribed.** Taking more methadone than prescribed can cause breathing to slow or stop and can cause death. A patient who does not experience good pain relief with the prescribed dose of methadone, should talk to his or her doctor. **2) Patients taking methadone should not start or stop taking other medicines or dietary supplements without talking to their health care provider.** Taking other medicines or dietary supplements may cause less pain relief. They may also cause a toxic buildup of methadone in the body leading to dangerous changes in breathing or heart beat that may cause death. **3) Health care professionals and patients should be aware of the signs of methadone overdose.** Signs of methadone overdose include trouble breathing or shallow breathing; extreme tiredness or sleepiness; blurred vision; inability to think, talk or walk normally; and feeling faint, dizzy or confused. If these signs occur, patients should get medical attention right away.

†Contains pellets of an extended-release oral formulation of morphine sulfate, an opioid receptor agonist, surrounding an inner core of naltrexone hydrochloride, an opioid receptor antagonist.

Appendix 14

Follow-Up Visit Form

Analgesia

If zero indicates "no pain" and 10 indicates "pain as bad as it can be," on a scale of 0 to 10, what is your level of pain for the following questions?

■ What was your pain level on average during the past week? (Please circle appropriate number.)

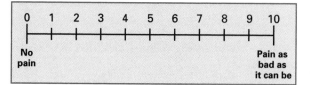

■ What was your pain level at its worst during the past week? (Please circle appropriate number.)

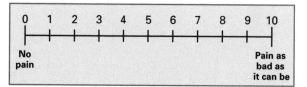

■ What percentage of your pain has been relieved during the past week? (Write in a percentage between 0% and 100%.)
_____%

■ Is the amount of pain relief you are now obtaining from your current pain reliever(s) enough to make a real difference?
❏ Yes ❏ No

Activities of Daily Living

■ Please indicate whether the patient's functioning with the current pain reliever(s) is better, the same, or worse since the patient's last assessment. (Please check the appropriate box for each item below.)

	Better	Same	Worse
Physical functioning	❏	❏	❏
Family relationships	❏	❏	❏
Social relationships	❏	❏	❏
Mood	❏	❏	❏
Sleep patterns	❏	❏	❏
Overall functioning	❏	❏	❏

Adverse Events

■ Is the patient experiencing any side effects from current pain relievers?
❏ Yes   ❏ No

■ Ask the patient about potential side effects:

	None	Mild	Moderate	Severe
Nausea	❏	❏	❏	❏
Vomiting	❏	❏	❏	❏
Constipation	❏	❏	❏	❏
Itching	❏	❏	❏	❏
Mental cloudiness	❏	❏	❏	❏
Sweating	❏	❏	❏	❏
Fatigue	❏	❏	❏	❏
Drowsiness	❏	❏	❏	❏
Reduced libido	❏	❏	❏	❏
Other	❏	❏	❏	❏

■ Patient's overall severity of side effects?
❏ None   ❏ Mild   ❏ Moderate   ❏ Severe

Addiction Behaviors Checklist

Check all behaviors that apply.

Addiction behaviors—since last visit
- ❑ Used illicit drugs or evidences problem drinking
- ❑ Has hoarded medications
- ❑ Used more opioid than prescribed
- ❑ Ran out of medications early
- ❑ Has increased use of opioids
- ❑ Used analgesics as needed when prescription is for time-contingent use
- ❑ Received opioids from more than one provider
- ❑ Bought medications on the streets

Addiction behaviors—within current visit
- ❑ Appears sedated or confused (e.g., slurred speech, unresponsive)
- ❑ Expresses worries about addiction
- ❑ Expresses a strong preference for a specific type of analgesic or a specific route of administration
- ❑ Expresses concern about future availability of opioid
- ❑ Reports worsened relationships with family
- ❑ Misrepresents analgesic prescription or use
- ❑ Indicates she or he "needs" or "must have" analgesic medications
- ❑ Requests office visit primarily to discuss analgesic medication
- ❑ Exhibits lack of interest in rehabilitation or self-management
- ❑ Reports minimal/inadequate relief from opioid
- ❑ Indicates difficulty with using patient medication agreement

Other
- ❑ Significant others express concern over patient's use of analgesics
- ❑ Other _____

Additional Studies/Tests

- ■ Urine medication monitoring (see Appendix 10)
  - ❑ Positive   ❑ Negative

  (Positive = presence of nonprescribed controlled medication, illicit substance, or alcohol)

■ Blood tests, including endocrine tests

_____

■ Prescription monitoring report (if available)
  ■ Indicates inappropriate behavior
  ■ Indicates appropriate behavior
  ■ Report not available

Comments: _____

_____

Assessment

■ COMM™ score (see Appendix 8)
  ■ Is your overall impression that this patient is benefiting from opioid (analgesic) therapy?
    ❑ Yes
    ❑ No
    ❑ Unsure

Comments: _____

_____

Action Plan

  ❑ Continue present opioid regimen
  ❑ Adjust regimen as follows:
    ❑ Add/adjust concomitant therapy
    ❑ Add/adjust nonpharmacologic therapy
    ❑ Adjust present opioid
    ❑ Rotate opioid
  ❑ Exit strategy: taper patient off opioid regimen
  ❑ Other:_____

Comments: _____

_____

Date:_____
Physician's signature: _____

Sources

Adapted from Pain Assessment and Documentation Tool (PADT™) courtesy of Steven Passik, PhD, Associate Attending Psychologist, Memorial Sloan-Kettering Cancer Center, New York, NY.

Checklist developed by Bruce D. Naliboff, PhD, with support from VA Health Services Research and Development. Used with permission.

Wu SM, Compton P, Bolus R, et al. The Addiction Behaviors Checklist: validation of a new clinician-based measure of inappropriate opioid use in chronic pain. *J Pain Symptom Manage* 2006;32:342–351.

Appendix 15

Opioid Conversion

Drug	Equianalgesic Dosage
Codeine	IM/IV/SC: 120 mg
	po: 200 mg
Fentanyl	0.1–0.2 mg
Hydrocodone	20–30 mg
Hydromorphone	IM/IV/SC: 1.3–1.5 mg
	po: 7.5 mg
Levorphanol	IM/IV/SC: 2 mg
	po: 4 mg
Meperidine*	IM/IV/SC: 75 mg
	po: 300 mg
Methadone	IM/IV/SC: 1–10 mg[†]
	Short-term: 5–10 mg
	Chronic use: 1–4 mg (2 mg)
	po: 2–20 mg[†]
	Short-term: 20 mg
	Chronic use: 2–4 mg (3 mg)
Morphine	IM/IV/SC: 10 mg
	po: 30–60 mg[‡]
Oxycodone	15–30 mg (20 mg)
Oxymorphone	IM/IV/SC: 1 mg
	po: 10 mg
Propoxyphene	130–200 mg[§]

IM = intramuscular; IV = intravenous; po = oral; SC = subcutaneous.

*Meperidine should be used for acute dosing only and not for chronic pain management (meperidine has a short half-life and a toxic metabolite: normeperidine). Its use should also be avoided in patients with renal insufficiency, chronic heart failure, hepatic insufficiency, or in the elderly because of the potential for toxicity due to accumulation of the metabolite normeperidine. Seizures, confusion, tremors, or mood alterations may be seen.

†Many equianalgesic tables underestimate methadone potency; more studies are needed. **Parenteral:** Program uses 10 mg for short-term dosing and 2 mg for chronic dosing. **Oral:** Program uses 20 mg for short-term dosing and 3 mg for chronic dosing.

‡**Acute dosing** (opiate-naive): 60 mg. **Chronic dosing:** 30 mg.

§**Propoxyphene HCL:** 130 mg; **Napsylate:** 200 mg (not recommended for chronic pain management and therefore not listed above).

Suggested Reading

McPherson, ML. *Demystifying Opioid Conversion Calculations: A Guide to Effective Dosing.* Bethesda, MD: American Society of Health-System Pharmacists; 2009.

Appendix 16

Exit Strategy for Discontinuing Opioid Therapy

- Determine risk-benefit ratio of continuation of opioid therapy considering factors including:
  - Intolerable side effects of effective dose
  - Reasonable unsuccessful attempts with opioid rotation
  - Poor compliance with mutually agreed upon opioid agreement
  - Controlled dose escalations without analgesic efficacy
  - Deterioration of quality of life related to opioid use
    - Physical function
    - Emotional state
    - Social interaction
- Promote shared decision-making with patient with regard to discontinuation of therapy
  - Review opioid agreement in detail
  - Reinforce the rationale (i.e., to benefit the patient)
  - Promote other therapeutic options
  - Reinforce that this is not abandonment
- Consider a variety of different scenarios with respect to opioid discontinuation, including:
  - **The patient has no apparent problems, and is able to comply with office-based tapering**
    - Taper opioid(s) gradually
    - Continue monitoring patient for aberrant behavior
    - Concurrently begin nonopioid strategies
      - ~ Nonopioid analgesics
      - ~ Psychosocial support
      - ~ Cognitive behavioral therapies
      - ~ Physical approaches
      - ~ Observation and management of dependence or pain-related symptoms

- Insomnia
- Anxiety
- Depression

■ **The patient appears to have signs and symptoms of addiction**
  - Refer for expert consultation or assistance with management

■ **The patient is unwilling or unable to cooperate with office-based tapering**
  - Provide sufficient opioid to bridge to transfer of management to an expert
  - Refer to inpatient or outpatient program as available

Appendix 17

Sample Patient Medication Agreement

The purpose of this agreement is to give you information about the medications you will be taking for pain management and to assure that you and your physician comply with all state and federal regulations concerning the prescribing of controlled substances. A trial of opioid therapy can be considered for moderate to severe pain with the intent of reducing pain and increasing function. The physician's goal is for you to have the best quality of life possible given the reality of your clinical condition. The success of treatment depends on mutual trust and honesty in the physician/patient relationship and full agreement with and understanding of the risks and benefits of using opioids to treat pain.

1. You should use **one** physician to prescribe and monitor all opioid medications and adjunctive analgesics.

2. You should use **one** pharmacy to obtain all opioid prescriptions and adjunctive analgesics prescribed by your physician.
   Pharmacy: _____
   Phone number: _____

3. You should inform your physician of all medications you are taking, including herbal remedies, as opioid medications can interact with over-the-counter medications and other prescribed medications, especially cough syrup that contains alcohol, codeine, or hydrocodone.

4. You will be seen on a regular basis and given prescriptions for enough medication to last from appointment to appointment, plus usually two to three days extra. This extra medication is **not** to be used without the explicit permission of the prescribing physician unless an emergency requires your appointment to be deferred one or two days.

5. Prescriptions for pain medicine or any other prescriptions will be done only during an office visit or during regular office hours. **No** refills of any medications will be done during the evening or on weekends.

6. You must bring back all opioid medications and adjunctive medications prescribed by your physician in the original bottles.

7. You are responsible for keeping your pain medication in a safe and secure place, such as a locked cabinet or safe. You are expected to protect your medications from loss or theft. Stolen medications should be reported to the police and to your physician immediately. If your medications are lost, misplaced, or stolen, your physician may choose not to replace the medications or to taper and discontinue the medications.

8. You may not give or sell your medications to any other person under any circumstances. If you do, you may endanger that person's health. It is also against the law.

9. Any evidence of drug hoarding, acquisition of any opioid medication or adjunctive analgesia from other physicians (which includes emergency rooms), uncontrolled dose escalation or reduction, loss of prescriptions, or failure to follow the agreement may result in termination of the doctor/patient relationship.

10. You will communicate fully to your physician to the best of your ability at the initial and all follow-up visits your pain level and functional activity along with any side effects of the medications. This information allows your physician to adjust your treatment plan accordingly.

11. You should not use any illicit substances, such as cocaine, marijuana, etc. while taking these medications. This may result in a change to your treatment plan, including safe discontinuation of your opioid medications when applicable or complete termination of the doctor/patient relationship.

12. The use of alcohol and opioid medications is contraindicated.

13. You agree and understand that your physician reserves the right to perform random or unannounced urine drug testing. If requested to provide a urine sample, you agree to cooperate. If you decide not to provide a urine sample, you understand that your doctor may change your treatment plan, including safe discontinuation of your opioid medications when applicable or complete termination of the doctor/patient relationship. The presence of a nonprescribed drug(s) or illicit drug(s) in the urine can be grounds for termination of the doctor/patient relationship. Urine drug testing is not forensic testing, but is done for your benefit as a diagnostic tool and in accordance with certain legal and regulatory materials on the use of controlled substances to treat pain.

14. There are side effects with opioid therapy, which may include, but not exclusively, skin rash, constipation, sexual dysfunction, sleeping abnormalities, sweating, edema, sedation, or the possibility of impaired cognitive (mental status) and/or motor ability. Overuse of opioids can cause decreased respiration (breathing).

15. Physical dependence and/or tolerance can occur with the use of opioid medications.

    Physical dependence means that if the opioid medication is abruptly stopped or not taken as directed, a withdrawal symptom can occur. This is a normal physiologic response. The withdrawal syndrome could include, but not exclusively, sweating, nervousness, abdominal cramps, diarrhea, goose bumps, and alterations in one's mood.

    It should be noted that physical dependence does not equal addiction. One can be dependent on insulin to treat diabetes or dependent on prednisone (steroids) to treat asthma, but one is not addicted to the insulin or prednisone.

    Addiction is a primary, chronic neurobiologic disease with genetic, psychosocial, and environmental factors influencing its development and manifestation. It is characterized by behavior that includes one or more of the following: impaired control over drug use, compulsive use, continued use despite harm, and cravings. This means the drug decreases one's quality of life.

Tolerance means a state of adaptation in which exposure to the drug induces changes that result in diminution of one or more of the drug's effects over time. The dose of the opioid may have to be titrated up or down to a dose that produces maximum function and a *realistic* decrease of the patient's pain.

16. If you have a history of alcohol or drug misuse/addiction, you must notify the physician of such history as the treatment with opioids for pain **may** increase the possibility of relapse. A history of addiction does not, in most instances, disqualify one for opioid treatment of pain, but starting or continuing a program for recovery is a must.

17. You agree to allow your physician to contact any health care professional, family member, pharmacy, legal authority, or regulatory agency to obtain or provide information about your care or actions *if the physician feels it is necessary.*

18. You agree to a family conference or a conference with a close friend or significant other *if the physician feels it is necessary.*

The above agreement has been explained to me by [INSERT PRESCRIBER NAME HERE]. I agree to its terms so that [INSERT PRESCRIBER NAME HERE] can provide quality pain management using opioid therapy to decrease my pain and increase my function.

Patient's Signature _____

Date _____

Witness's Signature _____

Date _____

"Agreement for Opioid Maintenance Therapy for Non-Cancer/Cancer Pain" provided courtesy of Howard A. Heit, MD, FACP, FASAM.
This agreement, as well as a Medication Management Agreement for patients with low literacy, can be downloaded at *http://www.PainEDU.org.*

Appendix 18

Internet Resources

General Pain Sites

PainEDU – *http://www.PainEDU.org*
painACTION – *http://www.painaction.com*
American Pain Society – *http://www.ampainsoc.org*

Laws or Legal Issues Regarding Opioid Treatment

Federation of State Medical Boards – *http://www.fsmb.org*
Drug Enforcement Administration, Office of Diversion Control –
    http://www.deadiversion.usdoj.gov
The Legal Side of Pain – *http://www.legalsideofpain.com*
University of Wisconsin Pain & Policy Studies Group – *http://
    www.painpolicy.wisc.edu*

Opioid Conversion Calculators

Epocrates – *http://www.epocrates.com*
GlobalRPh – *http://www.globalrph.com/narcoticonv.htm*
MedCalc – *http://www.medcalc.com*

Medication Safety

For patients – *http://www.painaction.com*
For clinicians – *http://www.PainEDU.org*

Risk Assessment Tools

PainEDU – *http://www.PainEDU.org*

Preventing and Managing Side Effects

For patients – *http://www.painaction.org*
For clinicians – *http://www.PainEDU.org*

Resources for Chronic Pain Patients

painACTION – *http://www.painaction.com*
American Chronic Pain Association – *http://www.theacpa.org*

Addiction Support Groups

Nar-Anon/Nar-Ateen – *http://www.nar-anon.org/Nar-Anon/
    Nar-Anon_Home.html*
Narcotics Anonymous (NA) – *http://www.na.org*
Partnership for a Drug-Free America – *http://www.drugfree.org*

References

1. Chou R, Fanciullo GJ, Fine PG, et al. Clinical guidelines for the use of chronic opioid therapy in chronic noncancer pain. *J Pain* 2009; 10(2):113–130.

2. Gammaitoni AR, Fine P, Alvarez N, et al. Clinical application of opioid equianalgesic data. *Clin J Pain* 2003;19:286–297.

3. Indelicato RA, Portenoy RK. Opioid rotation in the management of refractory cancer pain. *J Clin Oncol* 2002;20:348–352.

4. Quinn TE. Converting opioid analgesics, part I: use of equianalgesics tables. *Pain Relief Connection: The Pain Information Newsletter.* 2002;1:3–4.

5. American Pain Society. *Principles of Analgesic Use in the Treatment of Acute Pain and Cancer Pain.* 5th ed. Glenview, IL: American Pain Society; 2003.

6. U.S. Drug Enforcement Administration (DEA). *Supervisory Training: Guidelines for a Drug Free Workplace.* 4th ed. Alexandria, VA: U.S. Drug Enforcement Administration (DEA); 2003.

7. Wu SM, Compton P, Bolus R, et al. The addiction behaviors checklist: validation of a new clinician-based measure of inappropriate opioid use in chronic pain. *J Pain Symptom Manage* 2006;32:342–351.

8. Gourlay D, Heit H, Caplan Y. *Urine Drug Testing in Clinical Practice: Dispelling the Myths and Designing Strategies.* California Academy of Family Physicians Monograph. Stamford, CT: PharmaCom Group; 2004.

9. Brown RL, Leonard T, Saunders LA, Papasouliotis O. A two-item conjoint screen for alcohol and other drug problems. *J Am Board Fam Pract* 2001;14:95–106.

10. Delgin JH, Vallerand AH. *Davis's Drug Guide for Nurses.* 10th ed. Philadelphia: F. A. Davis; 2007.

11. *Physicians' Desk Reference.* 63rd ed. Montvale, NJ: Thomson Reuters; 2009.

12. Portenoy RK, Payne R, Passik SD. Acute and chronic pain. In: *Substance Abuse: A Comprehensive Textbook*, 4th ed. Philadelphia: Lippincott, Williams & Wilkins; 2005.